"Welcome to my book, "Discover the Potential of CBD: A Guide to Health Benefits". I'm thrilled that you're here and ready to deepen your knowledge of CBD.

This book is all about discovering the many health benefits of CBD and understanding how you can use them for yourself. I have thoroughly researched the topic and want to share all of my knowledge and experiences with you. You will find chapters in this book covering different applications of CBD, such as pain relief, sleep improvement, stress reduction, and even CBD use in sports.

This book is for anyone interested in the health benefits of CBD, whether you already have experience with CBD or are just getting started.

So, let's discover the potential of CBD together!

Best regards,

Rapha"

Disclaimer:

Please note that I am not a doctor and do not offer medical advice.

The information in this book is for general guidance only and should not be used as a substitute for medical advice or treatment.

If you have health problems, you should consult with a qualified medical professional.

The use of CBD and other complementary treatments should always be done in consultation with a medical professional."

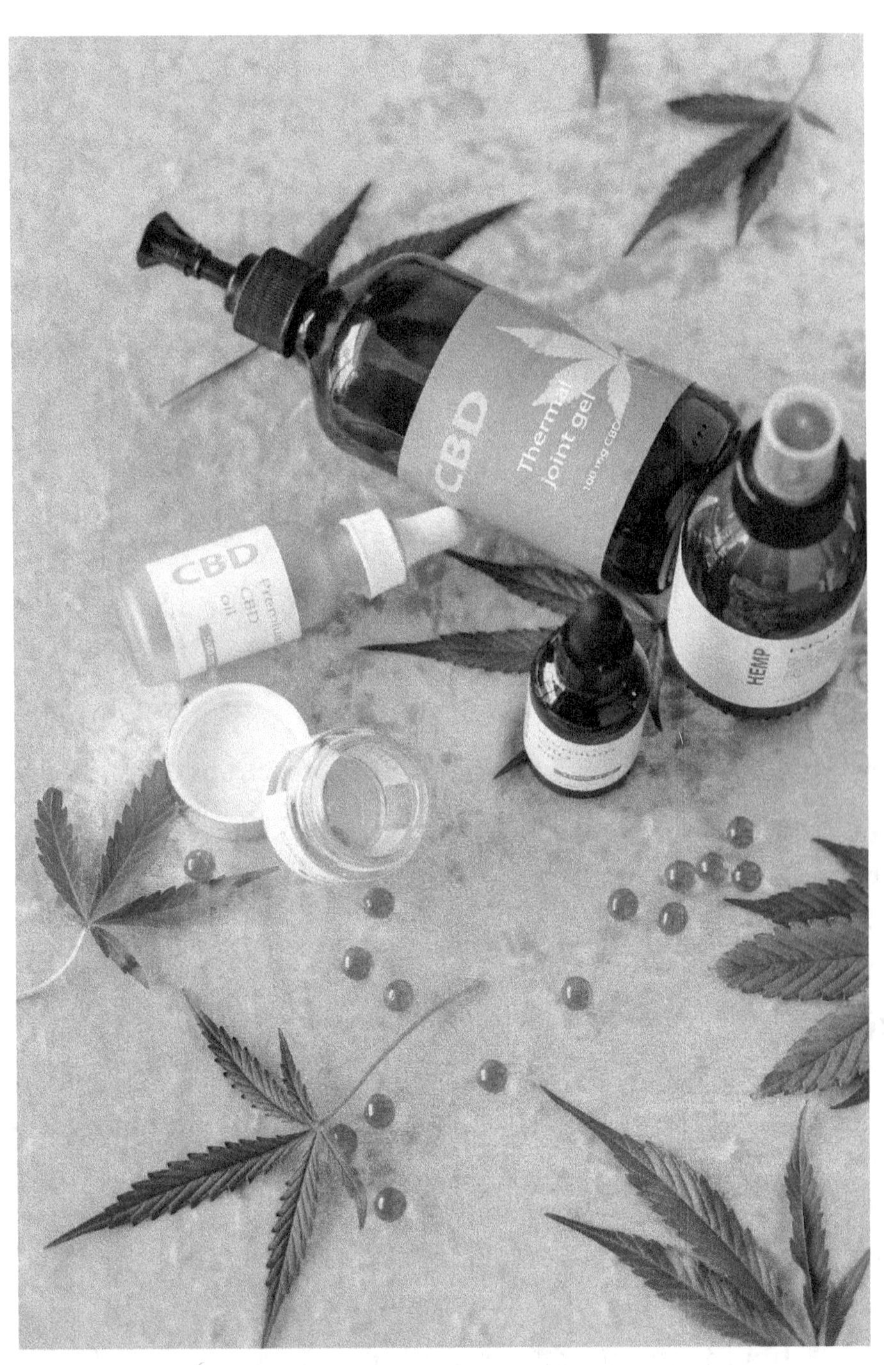

Pic by Nataliya Vaitkevic

Table of Contents:

Introduction to the book

Welcome to my book "Discover the Potential of CBD: A Guide to Health Benefits"! I'm excited that you're interested in this topic and ready to learn more.

CBD, or Cannabidiol, is a chemical compound extracted from the hemp plant. In recent years, CBD has gained popularity as it offers a variety of health benefits. However, with the abundance of information available on the internet, it can be difficult to discern what's true and what's not.

In this book, I'll provide you with a guide to the health benefits of CBD. I've compiled my knowledge and experience in this area to help you understand the science and research behind CBD and how it can contribute to improving your health. I'll also provide tips and advice for safe CBD use to ensure that you have the best possible experience.

However, I want to make it clear that I'm not a doctor or medical expert, and this book should not serve as a substitute for professional medical advice. If you have any questions or concerns about your health, I recommend consulting a doctor or healthcare professional before taking CBD or other supplements. The information contained in this book is intended as a guide to help you make the decision about whether CBD is right for you and how it can contribute to improving your health.

I hope this book helps you learn more about the benefits of CBD and how to use it safely and effectively. Thank you for choosing this book, and I hope you enjoy and find it useful!

Goals of the Book

The goal of this book is to introduce you to the world of CBD and help you understand and utilize the health benefits of CBD. I aim to provide you with clear and informative information about how CBD works, how it affects your body, and the positive impact it can have on your health.

I want to show you how to use CBD safely and effectively by presenting you with different methods of application and dosages. You will also learn about the potential side effects of CBD and how to minimize them.

In this book, we will focus on different areas of health where CBD can be helpful, such as sleep disorders, anxiety, pain, and inflammation. Additionally, we will explore the use of CBD in sports, as more and more athletes are turning to the potential benefits of CBD.

I want to emphasize that this book does not replace medical advice, and I am not a medical professional. I simply want to share my knowledge and experiences with you. Please always consult a doctor before taking CBD or other supplements.

My goal is for you to have a better understanding of CBD and how it can help improve your health after reading this book. I hope to provide you with a resource that will help you discover the benefits of CBD for yourself

<u>Target audience:</u>

I am writing this book primarily for people who want to learn more about the health benefits of CBD and who are curious about how to incorporate CBD products into their daily lives. This book is intended for anyone interested in a healthier and more natural lifestyle.

It is aimed at people who already use CBD products and want to deepen their knowledge, but also at beginners who have never heard of CBD or are skeptical about its effects. I want to encourage all readers to discover the health benefits of CBD and integrate them into their daily lives.

This book is not only for those interested in physical health, but also for those looking for ways to improve their mental health. CBD has a variety of benefits that can impact the well-being and health of the mind. In this book, we will discuss various CBD products that can have a positive impact on both physical and mental health.

I hope that this book appeals to people of all ages who are interested in a more natural lifestyle and who are curious about how CBD can help them. Whether you are young or old, athletic or not, this book provides you with all the necessary information to improve your health and well-being.

I hope that this book is a valuable source of information and inspiration for all readers, and that it helps to discover and utilize the many benefits of CBD.

What to expect from this book

As an avid proponent of natural healing methods, I have gained a lot of experience with CBD myself and now want to share this knowledge with you.

So, what can you expect from this book?

First and foremost, you will get a comprehensive overview of CBD and how it works in the body. I will explain the different forms of CBD products and how they are made. You will also learn about the potential health benefits of CBD and what research has been done in this area.

Furthermore, I will give you tips on how to use CBD and how to dose it properly. I will show you how CBD can help with various health problems and how it can be used as part of a holistic health strategy.

Another important aspect of the book is the use of CBD in sports. I will show you how CBD can help you recover faster, relieve pain, and improve your performance.

In addition to these practical application tips, there is also a lot of background knowledge on CBD, its history, and its role in society. You will understand why CBD is illegal in some countries and what political and economic factors play a role.

Overall, you can expect to gain a deeper understanding of CBD and its health benefits from this book. You will learn how to use CBD safely and effectively and how it can help you with various health problems. And last but not least, you will understand why CBD plays such an important role in today's society.

I hope you find this book as exciting and informative as I did when writing it.

What is CBD?

Introduction to the term CBD

CBD is short for cannabidiol, one of the many components found in the hemp plant. It is a natural, non-psychoactive molecule that is known for its versatile health-promoting properties. Unlike THC, another component found in hemp, CBD does not have intoxicating effects.

CBD can be consumed in various forms, including as oil, capsules, lotions, and even inhalation products. There are many studies that suggest CBD can be helpful in treating various conditions such as anxiety, depression, pain, and inflammation.

Difference between THC and CBD

As a CBD enthusiast, it's important to understand the difference between THC and CBD. THC and CBD are the two most well-known cannabinoids found in the cannabis plant. While THC is known for its psychoactive properties and has a intoxicating effect, CBD does not have psychoactive effects.

THC is the cannabinoid responsible for the "high" associated with smoking marijuana or consuming cannabis products. It also has some medical uses, such as relieving pain and reducing nausea. However, THC also has some undesirable effects, such as memory problems, anxiety, and paranoia.

CBD is a non-psychoactive cannabinoid that also occurs in the cannabis plant. It has many medical uses, such as reducing anxiety and depression, relieving pain and inflammation, and reducing seizures in epilepsy patients. CBD also has neuroprotective properties and can help in the treatment of neurodegenerative diseases such as Alzheimer's and Parkinson's.

While THC and CBD both come from the same plant, they have very different effects on the body. It's important to note that CBD products sold in Germany must have a THC content of less than 0.2%.

History and Development of CBD

As part of the cannabis plant, CBD has a long and fascinating history that goes back to the earliest days of human history. Thousands of years ago, various cultures recognized the therapeutic benefits of cannabis and used the plant for its medicinal properties.

In the modern Western world, scientists and researchers began identifying and studying the various components of cannabis in the 1940s. They discovered not only THC but also other cannabinoids such as CBD. In the 1960s, the structure of CBD was finally elucidated, and further investigations into the effects and benefits of CBD followed.

In the following decades, however, CBD increasingly fell into the background as the focus of scientists and researchers was on THC and its psychotropic effects. It wasn't until recent years that the potential of CBD as a therapeutic agent was rediscovered, and the research into the cannabinoid has experienced a true boom.

Today, CBD is legal in many parts of the world and is used for a variety of medical applications. In particular, in pain therapy, sleep disorders, anxiety, and inflammation, CBD has shown that it can be a promising active ingredient. CBD is also becoming increasingly important in the field of sports as a natural remedy for pain relief and regeneration.

Despite the growing popularity of CBD, there is still much to be explored and understood. However, the history and development of CBD show us that the research and use of the cannabis plant are a long-term project that continues to progress.

In this book, we will delve into the health benefits of CBD and help you discover the full potential of this fascinating compound.

CBD Extraction and Manufacturing

CBD products come in many forms and sizes, and it's important to understand how they are made to ensure you get a high-quality product. In the following, I will give you an insight into the process of CBD extraction and manufacturing.

First of all, CBD is extracted from the hemp plant. Hemp contains several compounds, including CBD and THC, but also many other cannabinoids, terpenes, flavonoids, and more. During CBD extraction, the goal is to isolate as much CBD as possible from the plant while minimizing THC to reduce its psychotropic effects.

There are different methods for extracting CBD, but the most common one is CO2 extraction. With this method, CO2 is passed through the hemp plant under high pressure and temperature to extract the cannabinoids and other compounds. The result is a highly concentrated CBD oil that can then be used for various purposes.

After extraction, the CBD oil undergoes a purification process to ensure it is free of impurities. It can also be diluted with carrier oils such as MCT oil or hemp seed oil to make dosing easier.

The quality of CBD oil depends on many factors, including the quality of the source material, the extraction process, and the purification process. It's important to buy a CBD product from a reputable manufacturer who provides detailed information about the manufacturing process.

CBD products can be made in various forms, including oil, capsules, tinctures, lotions, and more. Each form has its own advantages and disadvantages, depending on the consumer's needs. Some products act more quickly than others, while others have longer-lasting effects.

Overall, it's important to understand how CBD is made to ensure you get a high-quality product. The manufacturing process has a significant impact on the quality of the product and how it works, so it's important to choose a product that has been carefully and meticulously manufactured.

How does CBD affect our body?

<u>Introduction to the Endocannabinoid System (ECS)</u>

The Endocannabinoid System (ECS) is a complex network of receptors, enzymes, and molecules that play an important role in our body. It is closely connected to our nervous system, immune system, and many other systems in our body.

The ECS was first discovered in the 1990s when scientists were looking for an explanation for the effects of cannabis on the body. It turned out that the body is naturally able to produce cannabinoids, similar to the cannabinoids found in the hemp plant. These natural cannabinoids are called endocannabinoids.

The ECS is a system of receptors that respond to endocannabinoids as well as cannabinoids found in hemp and other plants. These receptors are found throughout the body, including the brain, nervous system, immune system, and digestive tract.

The ECS is capable of regulating many different functions in the body, including mood, appetite, sleep, pain, and inflammation. When the ECS is activated, it can help maintain homeostasis in the body by influencing various processes in the body.

Over the years, researchers have learned more about the ECS and how it relates to various aspects of health. It has been shown to play a role in regulating inflammation, pain, and supporting the immune system.

The ECS is an important part of the human body, and its significance for health is becoming increasingly clear. By using CBD, a cannabinoid derived from the hemp plant, we can activate the ECS and contribute to supporting our health.

In the next chapters, I will tell you more about how CBD and the ECS work together and how you can use CBD to support your health.

CBD and the ECS

CBD and the Endocannabinoid System (ECS) are closely linked. As I explained in the previous section, the ECS is a natural system in the body that plays an important role in regulating various bodily functions. The ECS consists of various parts, including cannabinoid receptors, endocannabinoids, and enzymes.

CBD affects the ECS by influencing the activity of cannabinoid receptors. CBD does not directly interact with the receptors, but rather indirectly by altering the activity of enzymes that normally break down endocannabinoids. When these enzymes are blocked, endocannabinoids can accumulate in the body and have a stronger effect on the cannabinoid receptors.

Through this interaction, CBD can offer various health benefits. For example, CBD can relieve pain by reducing pain perception and by inhibiting the activity of inflammatory mediators that cause pain and inflammation. CBD can also help regulate mood by inhibiting the breakdown of serotonin, a neurotransmitter that is important for regulating mood and sleep.

There is still much to be explored when it comes to the effects of CBD on the ECS, but it is clear that it is a promising connection. By learning more about the ECS and the interaction of CBD with it, you can better understand how CBD works and what benefits it can offer. In the next chapter, we will delve into some of the potential benefits of CBD for health.

CBD and Receptors in the Body

CBD interacts with the human body in various ways. One of the most important effects is its binding to specific receptors in the body that are part of the endocannabinoid system (ECS). The ECS includes a series of receptors and ligands that are present in the body and involved in regulating various processes.

There are two main types of cannabinoid receptors in the body, called CB1 and CB2 receptors. CB1 receptors are primarily found in the brain and central nervous system, while CB2 receptors are primarily located in peripheral tissues, including the immune system.

CBD does not directly interact with these receptors but influences them indirectly. CBD can slow down the breakdown of endocannabinoids in the body, making more endocannabinoids available for binding to CB1 and CB2 receptors. By enhancing the binding to these receptors, CBD can have a variety of effects on the body.

Another type of receptor that CBD can affect is serotonin receptors. Serotonin is a neurotransmitter responsible for regulating mood, sleep, and appetite. CBD can influence the effect of serotonin in the body, which may help reduce anxiety and depression.

Additionally, CBD can also interact with other receptors in the body, including the TRPV1 receptor, which is involved in regulating pain, inflammation, and body temperature, and the PPAR receptor, which is involved in regulating metabolism and inflammation.

Overall, the interaction of CBD with receptors in the body is complex and not yet fully understood. However, it is clear that CBD can have a variety of positive effects on the body by modulating the endocannabinoid system and interacting with other receptors in the body.

How CBD Works in the Body

W How does CBD work in the body? That's a question that many people are interested in, and in this chapter, I will try to answer it in as much detail as possible.

When CBD enters the body, it interacts with the endocannabinoid system (ECS), which plays an important role in maintaining balance in the body. The ECS consists of receptors that are distributed throughout the body, and endocannabinoids that the body produces itself.

CBD interacts with the ECS by modulating the activity of the receptors. Some studies have shown that CBD can inhibit the binding of endocannabinoids to the receptors, which can lead to an increase in their availability in the body. Other studies have shown that CBD can also influence the activity of other receptors, such as the serotonin receptors.

An important point is that CBD has no psychoactive effect. Unlike THC, which also interacts with the ECS but has a intoxicating effect, CBD has no impact on consciousness or perception.

However, the exact mechanisms of action of CBD in the body are still not fully understood, and there are many open questions that require further research. Some researchers believe that CBD may play a role in reducing inflammation and pain, while other studies have shown that CBD may also be effective in treating anxiety disorders and depression.

It is important to note that CBD is not a cure-all and that it may not be equally effective for all people. Each person has a unique ECS, and the effects of CBD can vary from person to person.

Overall, there is still much to discover when it comes to the effects of CBD in the body. But through the exploration of the endocannabinoid system and conducting studies, we can hopefully learn more about the many benefits of CBD.

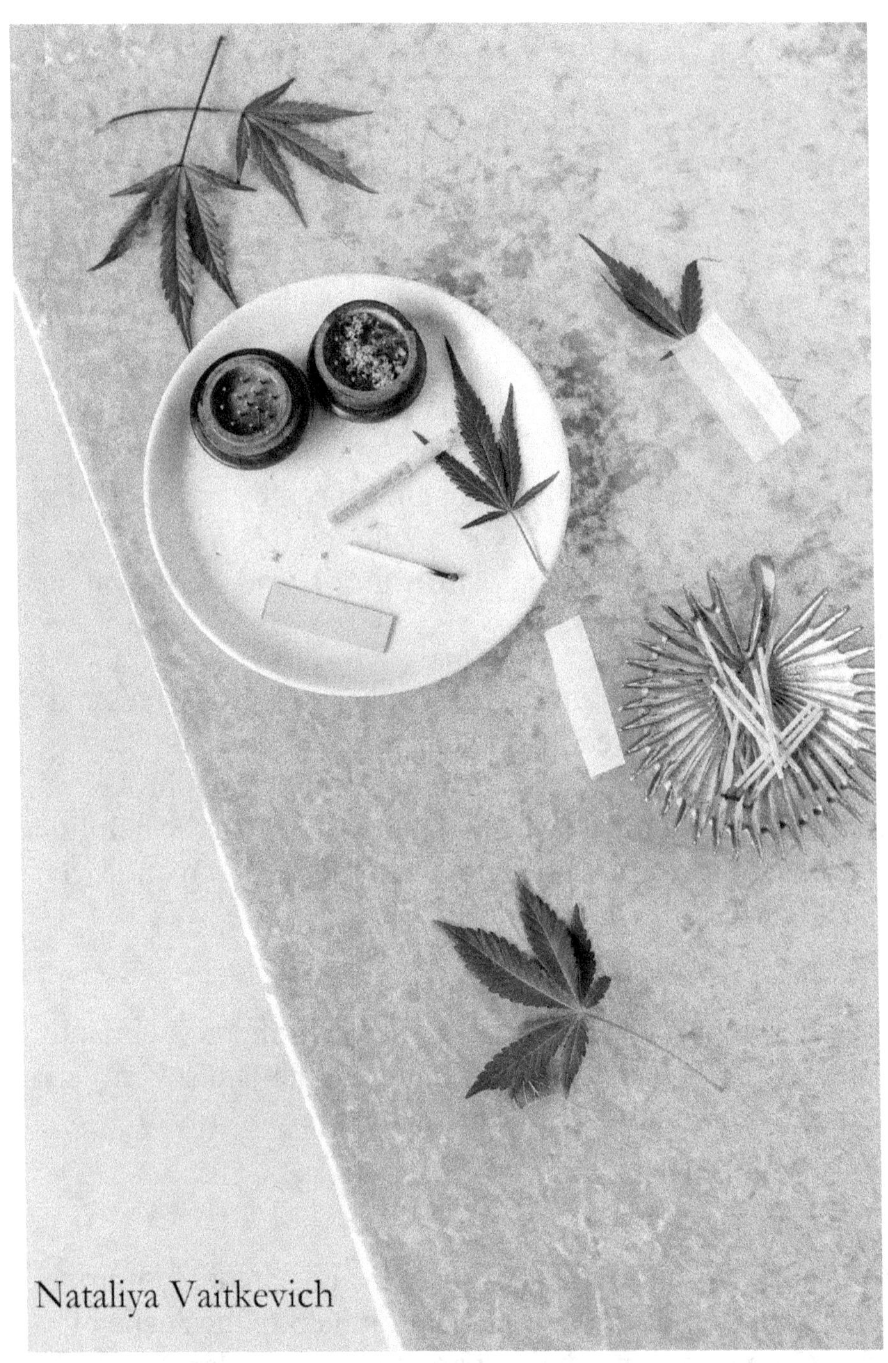

Nataliya Vaitkevich

<u>Introduction to the Benefits of CBD</u>

CBD has gained a lot of attention in recent years due to its potential health benefits. In this chapter, I'll give you an overview of the different benefits that CBD offers so that you can better understand how CBD can positively impact your health and well-being.

One of the most common uses of CBD is pain relief. Studies have shown that CBD has anti-inflammatory effects that can help alleviate pain caused by inflammation in the body. CBD can also help with the treatment of chronic pain such as back pain, arthritis, and fibromyalgia.

CBD also has a calming effect on the nervous system and can be helpful in treating anxiety and depression. It can help regulate serotonin levels in the brain and improve mood. Some studies have shown that CBD can be helpful in treating post-traumatic stress disorder (PTSD) and sleep disorders.

Another important use of CBD is the treatment of epileptic seizures. CBD can help reduce the number and severity of seizures, especially in children with severe forms of epilepsy such as Dravet syndrome.

CBD also has antioxidant properties and can help improve the health of the skin and hair. It can help reduce acne by regulating sebum production and reducing inflammation in the body. CBD can also help promote hair growth and improve hair health.

Finally, CBD can also be helpful in the treatment of addiction. It can help reduce withdrawal symptoms and decrease the craving for addictive substances.

There are many other potential benefits of CBD, including the treatment of diabetes, autoimmune diseases, and cancer. However, research in this area is still ongoing, and more studies need to be conducted to confirm these potential benefits.

Pain relief

CBD has proven to be a promising tool for pain relief and is already being used to treat chronic pain. Many studies have shown that CBD can help with pain relief by working in various ways in the body.

One of the ways in which CBD can alleviate pain is through its interaction with pain receptors in the body. CBD binds to these receptors and thereby inhibits the transmission of pain signals to the brain. This can effectively reduce pain and also have anti-inflammatory effects.

CBD has also been shown to influence the release of neurotransmitters responsible for pain regulation in the body. By taking CBD, the release of endorphins and serotonin can be increased, which can lead to an improved mood and a reduction in pain.

Another way in which CBD can help with pain relief is

through its anti-inflammatory properties. Chronic pain can be caused by inflammation in the body, and CBD can help reduce this inflammation. By reducing inflammation, pain can be significantly reduced, making it easier for people with chronic pain to cope with their daily lives.

There are many types of pain that CBD can be effective for, including headaches, joint pain, back pain, and neuropathic pain. In a study of people with multiple sclerosis, CBD was found to significantly reduce pain and improve mobility.

CBD also has the potential to enhance the pain relief of other medications. A study from 2010 showed that CBD in combination with opioids can help enhance pain relief and reduce the amount of opioid dosage required. This can help reduce the negative side effects of opioids, such as dependence.

In summary, CBD can help with pain relief in various ways, including through its interaction with pain receptors, influence on neurotransmitters, and anti-inflammatory properties. CBD has the potential to be effective for many types of pain and can also enhance the pain relief of other medications. If you are experiencing pain, CBD may be a promising option for finding relief.

Anxiety and Stress Reduction

CBD has gained a lot of attention in recent years as a potential remedy for anxiety and stress. Its calming effect on the nervous system and its ability to lower cortisol levels in the body make it a promising tool for addressing these common issues.

Stress is an unavoidable part of modern life. Many people feel stressed and overwhelmed, which can lead to physical and mental health problems. A common result of stress is the release of the hormone cortisol, which can have inflammatory effects at high doses and can also impair the immune system.

CBD can help calm the nervous system and lower cortisol levels. Studies have shown that CBD can help reduce anxiety and stress, improve sleep, and stabilize mood.

CBD can also be helpful in treating anxiety disorders such as generalized anxiety disorder, social anxiety disorder, post-traumatic stress disorder (PTSD), and obsessive-compulsive disorder. A 2015 study found that CBD may be more effective than conventional medications such as benzodiazepines in treating anxiety disorders.

Another benefit of CBD in addressing anxiety and stress is its ability to reduce inflammation in the body. Chronic inflammation is associated with many health problems, including depression and anxiety. CBD can reduce inflammation in the body and contribute to improving mental health.

CBD can be taken in various forms, including oils, capsules, gummies, and topical products. Each type of product has its own benefits and may be suitable for different situations and needs.

However, it is important to be aware that CBD is not suitable for everyone and that there may be possible side effects such as fatigue, nausea, and diarrhea. It is also important to talk to a doctor before taking CBD, especially if you are already taking medications or have a chronic condition.

Overall, CBD is a promising option for addressing anxiety and stress. It has a calming effect on the nervous system and can help reduce inflammation, which may contribute to improving mental health. If you are considering using CBD as an alternative or supplement to traditional treatment methods, talk to a doctor to determine if it is right for you.

Improving Sleep with CBD

CBD is increasingly being used as a sleep aid. There is a growing body of research that shows CBD can improve the quality of sleep. But how does it work?

The endocannabinoid system (ECS) plays an important role in regulating sleep. The ECS is a complex network of receptors, enzymes, and endocannabinoids that all contribute to maintaining the body's balance. The main function of the ECS is to maintain the balance of the body's various systems. When the ECS is not functioning properly, it can lead to sleep disturbances.

CBD has been shown to influence the activity of the ECS. It can increase the number of endocannabinoids in the body and activate the receptors involved in regulating sleep. CBD can also regulate the release of hormones and neurotransmitters that affect sleep.

One of the main causes of sleep disturbances is stress and anxiety. CBD has been shown to reduce stress and anxiety, which in turn can improve sleep. When one is less stressed and feels more relaxed, it is easier to fall asleep and stay asleep.

Another way that CBD can improve sleep is by reducing pain and inflammation. Pain and inflammation can make it harder to fall asleep and stay asleep. CBD has been shown to reduce pain and inflammation, which can improve sleep.

A study published in the Journal of Clinical Psychology showed that CBD reduced symptoms of anxiety and sleep disturbances in patients with post-traumatic stress disorder (PTSD). Another study published in the Journal of Psychopharmacology showed that CBD increased total sleep time in patients with sleep disorders.

Improvement of Mood

CBD has the potential to improve mood and reduce emotional instability. It is known that CBD has a direct effect on the brain and nervous system, and thus can regulate mood.

A study published in the journal "CNS & Neurological Disorders - Drug Targets" in 2019 examined the effect of CBD on mood. The study found that CBD can help alleviate symptoms and improve mood in patients with anxiety disorders and depression. CBD has been identified as a potentially effective treatment for various mental disorders such as anxiety, depression, and post-traumatic stress disorder.

One possible explanation for the effect of CBD on mood is its ability to increase serotonin levels in the brain. Serotonin is a neurotransmitter responsible for regulating mood and well-being. CBD can increase the level of serotonin in the brain through its interactions with the ECS, which can lead to a feeling of relaxation and mood improvement.

In addition, CBD also has anti-inflammatory and antioxidant properties that can help reduce stress and inflammation in the body. Stress and inflammation are known to be associated with a poor mood, so the ability of CBD to reduce stress and inflammation can contribute to an improvement in mood.

Overall, CBD is a promising way to improve mood and reduce emotional instability. There are numerous studies suggesting that CBD may be effective in treating anxiety, depression, and other mental disorders. If you suffer from any of these conditions or simply want to improve your mood, CBD can be a useful addition to your routine.

Improving Skin Health

The skin is the largest organ in the body and has many important functions, including protecting against external factors such as dirt, bacteria, and UV radiation. It is also an important part of the immune system and helps to protect the body from infections. Therefore, having healthy skin is crucial for our overall health and well-being.

CBD can help improve skin health in various ways. One way is that it possesses anti-inflammatory properties that can help reduce inflammation and soothe the skin. Inflammation can lead to various skin problems such as acne, eczema, rosacea, and psoriasis, and CBD can help alleviate these issues.

Another way CBD can contribute to improving skin health is that it is a potent antioxidant. Antioxidants can help combat free radicals in the body that can cause damage to the skin. CBD can thus help protect the skin from damage caused by UV radiation, environmental pollution, and other external factors.

CBD can also help regulate the skin's moisture balance. Healthy skin requires moisture to stay supple and elastic. CBD can help regulate the skin's moisture balance by regulating sebum production. Excessive sebum production can lead to oily skin and acne, while insufficient sebum production can lead to dry skin.

Another way CBD can contribute to improving skin health is that it can help in the healing of skin injuries and conditions. It can help speed up the healing of cuts, burns, abrasions, and other injuries. It can also help alleviate skin conditions such as eczema and psoriasis by reducing inflammation and relieving itchiness.

CBD can be applied to the skin in various ways, including topical applications such as creams, lotions, and salves. It can also be taken in the form of CBD oils, which can be ingested orally or applied directly to the skin.

Overall, CBD can contribute to improving skin health due to its anti-inflammatory, antioxidant, and moisturizing properties. If you suffer from skin problems or simply want to improve your skin health, CBD could be a natural and effective option to help you achieve your goal.

Reduction of Inflammation

Inflammation is a natural defense mechanism of the body against harmful stimuli. It is a complex physiological reaction triggered by various messenger molecules and immune cells. However, there are also chronic inflammations that can lead to various diseases. CBD can help reduce inflammation in the body.

CBD has anti-inflammatory properties that can work in several ways. On the one hand, it can reduce the production of pro-inflammatory cytokines that are involved in the development of inflammation. On the other hand, CBD can modulate the activity of immune cells by inhibiting the recruitment of inflammation cells and the release of inflammation factors.

Studies have shown that CBD can help with various inflammatory diseases, such as arthritis, inflammatory bowel disease, neurological inflammation, and even skin inflammation. CBD can also help with inflammation after injuries and surgeries.

Another way CBD can help with inflammation is its ability to reduce oxidative stress. Oxidative stress is an imbalance between the production of reactive oxygen species and the body's ability to break them down. This can lead to damage to cells and tissues and promote inflammation. CBD can help reduce oxidative stress through its antioxidant properties and thus prevent inflammation.

In summary, CBD can be a promising remedy for treating inflammation in the body due to its anti-inflammatory properties. It can reduce the production of inflammation factors, modulate the activity of immune cells, reduce oxidative stress, and thus prevent or alleviate inflammation.

Reduction of Nausea and Vomiting

Nausea and vomiting are two symptoms that can have a variety of causes, including illness, chemotherapy, or motion sickness. While there are various treatment options available, many people have chosen to use CBD for reducing nausea and vomiting.

Studies have shown that CBD can affect activity in the brain, particularly in the area of the vomiting center, which can lead to relief from nausea and vomiting. In fact, CBD has been particularly effective in reducing nausea and vomiting associated with chemotherapy.

A 2016 study examined the effects of CBD on nausea and vomiting in patients undergoing chemotherapy. Participants were given a combination of THC and CBD or a placebo. The study found that the combination of THC and CBD was significantly more effective in reducing nausea and vomiting than the placebo.

There is also evidence to suggest that CBD may help reduce nausea and vomiting associated with other conditions such as Crohn's disease and ulcerative colitis. A 2013 study examined the effects of CBD on rats with intestinal inflammation. The study found that CBD significantly reduced the severity of symptoms, including nausea and vomiting.

It is important to note that CBD should be used as a supplement to other treatments for reducing nausea and vomiting. If you have persistent nausea and vomiting, you should consult a doctor to investigate the underlying cause and receive appropriate treatment.

Other potential benefits of CBD

CBD has a variety of potential benefits that have been studied in different research studies. In this chapter, I will discuss some of the other possible benefits of CBD.

A promising application of CBD is its potential effect on the cardiovascular system. CBD has been shown to lower blood pressure and may also help reduce inflammation in the heart. A 2017 study showed that CBD reduced damage to blood vessels caused by high blood sugar levels. Another study in 2018 found that CBD reduced damage to heart muscle caused by a heart attack. However, further research is needed to clarify how exactly CBD affects the cardiovascular system and which doses and forms of intake are best suited.

CBD also has the potential to help in the treatment of diabetes. A 2016 study found that CBD could regulate insulin production and blood sugar levels in mice. Another study in 2018 showed that CBD reduced inflammation in pancreatic tissue and increased insulin production. Again, further research is needed to determine how effective CBD can be in treating diabetes in humans.

Other potential applications of CBD include the treatment of addiction and mental illnesses such as schizophrenia and epilepsy. A 2019 study found that CBD could help reduce alcohol consumption and relapse in alcohol addiction. Another study in 2018 showed that CBD reduced symptoms of schizophrenia and improved cognitive function. And there is also increasing evidence that CBD can be effective in treating epilepsy and other seizure disorders.

Finally, there is also evidence that CBD could help in the treatment of cancer and other serious illnesses. A 2018 study found that CBD can help inhibit the growth of tumor cells and slow the spread of cancer cells. Another study in 2019 showed that CBD can inhibit the growth of breast cancer cells.

It is important to emphasize that these potential benefits of CBD require further research to fully understand how and why CBD affects the body. It is also important to note that CBD should not be used as a substitute for proper medical treatment. If you have a medical condition, you should always consult a doctor and not rely solely on CBD to treat your symptoms.

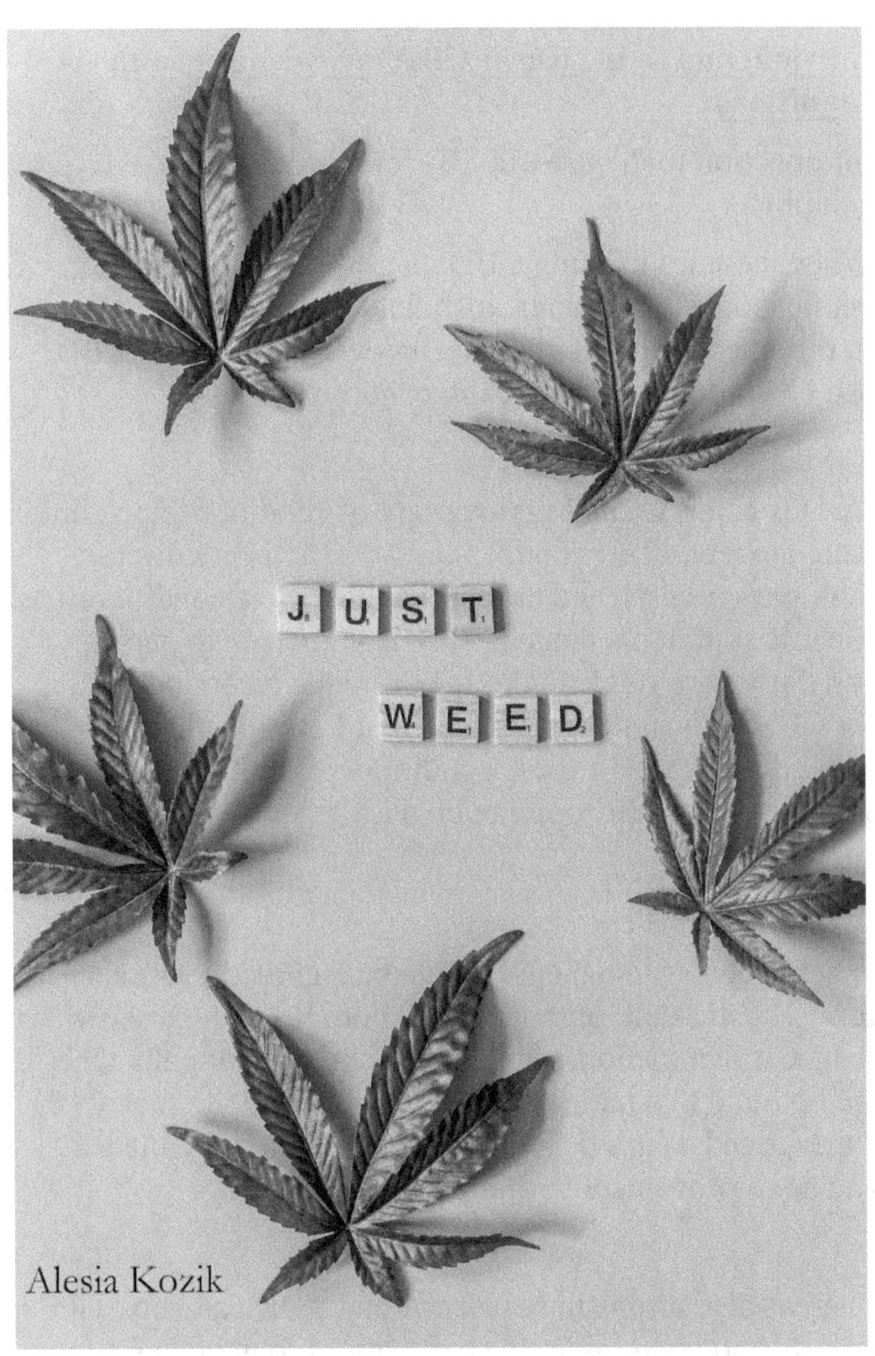

Alesia Kozik

Introduction to the use of CBD for various health conditions

Introduction to the use of CBD for various health conditions

When it comes to using CBD, there are many potential applications, but it can be difficult to know where to start. In this chapter, I will give you an overview of how CBD can be used for various health conditions.

CBD is being studied for a variety of conditions, including pain, anxiety, depression, epilepsy, Parkinson's disease, multiple sclerosis, and cancer. Each of these conditions has specific symptoms that can vary from person to person, and there is no uniform dosage or intake recommendation for CBD. It is important to note that CBD should not be viewed as a cure for these conditions, but rather as an aid that can be used in conjunction with other treatments and lifestyle changes.

When it comes to pain, CBD can be applied in various forms, such as oil, ointment, or lotion. It has been shown to reduce inflammation, which can be helpful for pain. One study found that patients with chronic pain who took CBD experienced a significant reduction in their pain intensity and an improvement in their sleep quality.

There is also promising evidence that CBD can help with anxiety and depression. In study, it was found that CBD reduced anxiety symptoms in patients with social anxiety disorder. Another study found that CBD can help reduce the occurrence of negative thoughts in patients with depression.

For epilepsy patients, there is already an approved medication called Epidiolex that contains CBD. It has been approved for the treatment of two rare forms of epilepsy and has proven to be effective. In a clinical study, patients who took Epidiolex experienced a significant reduction in the number of seizures.

Parkinson's disease patients have also benefited from the use of CBD. One study found that CBD can reduce the occurrence of Parkinson's symptoms such as tremors and restlessness.

People with multiple sclerosis have also shown positive results from using CBD. It has been shown to reduce spasticity, which is a major problem for many MS patients. One study found that CBD significantly reduced muscle stiffness and pain in MS patients.

Regarding cancer, studies have shown that CBD can help reduce nausea and vomiting caused by chemotherapy. There is also evidence that CBD can inhibit the growth of cancer cells, but further research is needed to confirm this.

These are just a few examples of the use of CBD for various health conditions. More information will be provided in the next chapters.

CBD and Pain

CBD has the potential to relieve pain and is being investigated in many studies as a promising treatment option for various types of pain. Pain can be caused by a variety of conditions and states, such as chronic pain due to arthritis or fibromyalgia, neuropathic pain due to nerve damage, pain due to cancer or chemotherapy, as well as pain due to injuries or surgeries.

CBD interacts with our endocannabinoid system, which plays an important role in pain perception. It can help relieve pain by reducing inflammation and blocking the pain receptor. It can also influence pain perception by affecting the neurotransmitters involved in the transmission of pain signals.

A 2018 study published in the Journal of Headache and Pain examined the effects of CBD on people with migraines. The study found that CBD may be effective as a prophylactic treatment for migraines, as it reduces the frequency of migraine attacks and relieves pain during an attack.

Another study from 2015 examined the effects of Sativex, a medication containing THC and CBD, on people with multiple sclerosis. The study found that Sativex significantly reduced pain in people with multiple sclerosis and improved their sleep quality.

CBD can also be helpful in treating neuropathic pain caused by nerve damage. A 2019 study published in the

Journal of Pain Research found that CBD can reduce pain in patients with neuropathic pain who did not respond to other treatment options.

CBD is also a promising treatment option for pain related to cancer. A 2010 study published in the Journal of Pain and Symptom Management found that CBD significantly reduced pain in patients with advanced cancer who did not respond to other pain medications.

However, it is important to note that CBD is not a universal solution for pain and that the effects of CBD on pain can vary from person to person.

CBD and Anxiety

Anxiety can be a very unpleasant experience and can affect various aspects of your life. It can impact your work, relationships, and overall quality of life. Many people are looking for natural ways to relieve their symptoms, and CBD is increasingly being considered as a possible solution. In this chapter, I will explain how CBD can help alleviate anxiety.

Firstly, it is important to understand what anxiety is. It occurs when your body enters a survival response, often referred to as "fight or flight." When your brain believes there is a threat, it releases a flood of hormones, including adrenaline and cortisol. These hormones increase your heart rate, breathing, and muscle tension to prepare you to either fight or flee. Anxiety can occur during this response. However, if the threat is not actually physical, it can be difficult to stop this response, leading to persistent anxiety.

One way to alleviate anxiety is to interrupt or reduce this survival response in the body. CBD has the potential to do this by interacting with the endocannabinoid system (ECS), a complex network of receptors and neurotransmitters responsible for a variety of body functions, including the regulation of mood, appetite, and sleep. CBD has an affinity for CB1 receptors in the central nervous system responsible for regulating anxiety and mood. A 2019 clinical study found that CBD reduced activity in areas of the brain responsible for assessing threats and triggering anxiety.

There is also evidence that CBD can lower the level of the stress hormone cortisol in the body. A 2019 study found that CBD reduced cortisol production and participants in the study reported feeling less stressed. This could help alleviate the body's survival response to threats.

However, it is important to note that not all studies have shown positive results. Some research has found that CBD can actually worsen anxiety in some people. It is unclear why this is the case, and further research is needed to better understand the effects of CBD on anxiety.

CBD and Sleep Disorders

One of the biggest benefits of CBD is its ability to improve sleep. Many people suffer from sleep disorders, whether it's insomnia, sleep apnea, or other causes. If you're one of these people, CBD could be a natural solution to help you sleep better.

As we've discussed, CBD interacts with the endocannabinoid system, which is involved in regulating the sleep-wake cycle. Studies have shown that CBD can help treat sleep disorders by prolonging overall sleep time and reducing the likelihood of waking up during the night.

Some research suggests that CBD may also be helpful in treating sleep apnea, a common condition where breathing stops during sleep. It's believed that CBD reduces inflammation that can cause breathing problems, leading to an improvement in sleep quality.

If you want to use CBD to improve your sleep, there are various ways to take it. CBD oils and capsules can be a good choice as they're easy to dose and typically take effect within 20 to 30 minutes. There are also specific CBD products designed for sleep, such as CBD sleep drops or CBD sleep tablets.

If you choose CBD oil, take it about 30 minutes before bedtime to achieve maximum effect. Start with a low dose and increase it slowly until you achieve the desired effect. It's important to ensure that you're buying high-quality CBD products to ensure that you're getting an effective and safe solution for your sleep disorders.

It's also important to note that CBD doesn't work the same for everyone. Some people may experience a quick improvement in their sleep disorders, while others may take longer to see an effect. If you're taking CBD regularly and not seeing an improvement in your sleep quality, talk to a doctor to discuss other options.

CBD and Depression

Depression is a common mental illness that affects millions of people worldwide. The symptoms can be very severe, ranging from sadness and hopelessness to thoughts of suicide. Although there are many treatment options, not all patients respond to them or experience unpleasant side effects. However, there is growing evidence that CBD may be a promising option for the treatment of depression.

As we have already discussed, CBD can help improve mood by increasing serotonin production in the brain. Serotonin is an important neurotransmitter involved in the regulation of mood. A 2014 study found that CBD can stimulate the production of serotonin in the brain, thereby improving mood. In addition, another 2018 study found that CBD can improve mood in people with anxiety disorders, which is a common feature of depression.

There is also evidence that CBD has an anti-inflammatory effect that can help combat inflammation in the brain associated with depression. A 2019 study showed that CBD had an anti-inflammatory effect in rats with depression and also helped improve their mood.

In another 2018 study, CBD was examined as a potential treatment option for patients with severe depression. The study found that CBD was safe and well-tolerated and also resulted in a significant improvement in symptoms. Although further research in this area is needed, the results are promising.

However, it is important to note that CBD alone is not a complete treatment for depression. A comprehensive treatment typically requires a combination of different therapies and/or medications. If you are suffering from depression, it is important to speak with a qualified healthcare provider to receive appropriate treatment.

If you are considering using CBD for the treatment of depression, it is important to choose a high-quality CBD product. Make sure the product comes from a reputable brand and has been tested for purity and potency by a third-party laboratory. As with any supplement or medication, it is also important to follow the manufacturer's dosage recommendations and speak with a qualified healthcare provider if necessary.

CBD and Acne

When it comes to skincare, acne can be one of the most burdensome conditions. Acne is an inflammatory skin condition caused by an overproduction of sebum. This can lead to clogged pores that become inflamed and result in pimples and blackheads. While there are many products that can help treat acne, they can often be expensive and contain a lot of chemicals.

CBD is a natural option that can help in the treatment of acne. It has been shown to have anti-inflammatory properties, meaning it can reduce inflammation in the body. When it comes to acne, CBD can help reduce inflammation in the affected areas and alleviate symptoms.

A 2014 study looked at the effects of CBD on sebaceous glands and found that CBD is able to inhibit sebum production. This is an important factor in the development of acne, as overproduction of sebum can lead to clogged pores and inflammation. By inhibiting sebum production, CBD can help reduce the occurrence of acne.

Another study from 2016 looked at the effects of CBD on inflammation and found it to be effective in reducing inflammation in various areas of the body. Although this study did not specifically target acne, it is likely that CBD is also helpful in reducing inflammation related to acne.

CBD can also help soothe and hydrate the skin, which can help reduce the occurrence of acne. When the skin is dry, it may tend to produce more sebum, which can worsen the occurrence of acne. By moisturizing the skin, CBD can help regulate sebum production and reduce the occurrence of acne.

When it comes to using CBD for the treatment of acne, there are a variety of options. One option is to use topical CBD products that can be applied to the affected areas. There are also CBD oils that can be taken orally to achieve an anti-inflammatory effect throughout the body.

CBD and Inflammation

Inflammation is an important part of the body's defense mechanism, but it can also be a symptom of many diseases. Pain, swelling, and redness are the typical signs of inflammation, triggered by an overproduction of pro-inflammatory molecules such as cytokines and interleukins.

CBD has shown potential as a means of reducing inflammation by acting on various signaling pathways in the body. CBD can inhibit the production of pro-inflammatory molecules and increase the production of anti-inflammatory molecules.

An important signaling pathway that CBD affects is the endocannabinoid system (ECS) in the body. The ECS is a network of receptors and messenger molecules involved in regulating functions such as inflammation, pain, mood, and appetite. CBD interacts with the receptors of the ECS, thereby influencing the release of neurotransmitters and hormones involved in the inflammatory response.

A 2012 study examined the effects of CBD on inflammation and pain in rats. The researchers found that CBD significantly reduced inflammation in the animals by inhibiting the release of pro-inflammatory cytokines.

Another 2016 study examined the effects of CBD on inflammatory skin conditions such as psoriasis. The researchers found that CBD reduced inflammation in skin tissue by inhibiting the activity of certain pro-inflammatory enzymes.

CBD has also shown effectiveness in treating inflammatory bowel diseases such as Crohn's disease and ulcerative colitis. A 2011 study found that CBD reduced inflammation and damage in the intestinal tissue of rats by inhibiting the release of pro-inflammatory molecules.

Another 2018 study examined the effects of CBD on ulcerative colitis in humans. The researchers found that CBD significantly reduced the clinical symptoms of the disease and reduced inflammation in the intestinal tissue.

CBD may also be effective in relieving inflammation associated with neurodegenerative diseases such as Alzheimer's, Parkinson's, and multiple sclerosis. A 2015 study found that CBD reduced inflammation and damage in the brains of rats with Alzheimer's.

Overall, research suggests that CBD may be a promising means of reducing inflammation.

CBD and Nausea/Vomiting

When it comes to the use of CBD, there are many potential benefits to consider. One of the most promising applications of CBD is the relief of nausea and vomiting. In this chapter, we will delve deeper into how CBD works in the body to combat these symptoms, as well as the current research and possible applications.

Nausea and vomiting are symptoms that can be caused by a variety of health conditions, including cancer, chemotherapy, motion sickness, pregnancy, and many others. It can be difficult to effectively treat these symptoms, as conventional medications often have unwanted side effects and are not always effective. However, CBD has proven to be a promising alternative.

CBD works in the body by interacting with the endocannabinoid system. This system is a network of receptors and neurotransmitters that play an important role in regulating a variety of bodily functions, including mood, appetite, pain perception, and nausea. CBD works on this system by activating the receptors and regulating the release of neurotransmitters, which can contribute to the relief of nausea and vomiting.

Research on CBD and nausea/vomiting is promising. A 2011 study found that CBD reduced the effects of chemotherapy-induced nausea and vomiting in rats. Another study in 2014 found that CBD could reduce nausea and vomiting in patients undergoing chemotherapy. Although further research is necessary to understand the exact mechanisms of action, CBD appears to be a promising means of relieving nausea and vomiting.

There are various ways to use CBD for the relief of nausea and vomiting. One way is to use CBD oils, which can be ingested orally or used in foods and beverages. Another way is to use CBD capsules or tablets, which can be ingested orally. There are also topical CBD products that can be applied to the skin to relieve nausea and vomiting.

It is important to note that the dosage of CBD for the relief of nausea and vomiting varies depending on individual needs. It is advisable to start with a low dose and gradually increase the dose until the desired effect is achieved. It is also important to consult with a qualified doctor before using CBD for the relief of nausea and vomiting, especially if you are taking other medications or are pregnant.

<u>**Other Applications of CBD**</u>

CBD, or cannabidiol, is a fascinating substance with a wide range of potential applications. In this chapter, I will discuss some of these applications that have not been covered in detail thus far.

One potential application of CBD that is being studied in research is its effect on the cardiovascular system. Some studies have shown that CBD can lower blood pressure and reduce heart rate. This could potentially be a promising treatment option for people with high blood pressure or other cardiovascular conditions. However, further studies are necessary to confirm these effects and to clarify exactly how CBD works on the cardiovascular system.

Another promising application of CBD is its effect on the immune system. CBD has immunomodulatory properties, which means that it can influence the function of the immune system. In animal studies, it has been shown that CBD can reduce inflammation and regulate the immune system. These effects could be useful in the treatment of autoimmune diseases such as multiple sclerosis and rheumatoid arthritis.

CBD may also play a role in the treatment of addiction. There is evidence that CBD may help alleviate withdrawal symptoms in people with alcohol or drug addiction. One study found that CBD was able to reduce anxiety and impulsivity in people with heroin addiction. However, further studies are necessary to confirm these effects and to clarify exactly how CBD works on withdrawal symptoms.

Another promising application of CBD is its potential effect on the nervous system. There is evidence that CBD could be beneficial in the treatment of neurodegenerative diseases such as Alzheimer's and Parkinson's. In animal studies, it has been shown that CBD can help alleviate the symptoms of these diseases and reduce the development of nerve cell damage. However, further studies are necessary to confirm these effects and to clarify exactly how CBD works on the nervous system.

Another promising application of CBD is its effect on bone metabolism. In animal studies, it has been shown that CBD can contribute to promoting bone formation and accelerating bone healing. This could potentially be a promising treatment option for people with bone diseases such as osteoporosis. However, further studies are necessary to confirm these effects and to clarify exactly how CBD works on bone metabolism.

CBD for pets

Introduction to using CBD for animals

The use of CBD for animals is becoming increasingly popular as more and more pet owners discover the potential benefits of CBD for their pets. If you're considering using CBD for your pet, it's important to educate yourself on its application, dosage, and potential benefits and risks.

CBD can be used for animals in similar ways as for humans. There are many different products on the market that are suitable for animals, such as oils, treats, capsules, and salves. It's important to choose a product that has been specifically formulated for animals and does not contain any ingredients that may be toxic to them.

There is no universal rule for dosing CBD for animals, as every dog or cat is different. Dosage depends on factors such as weight, age, health condition, and severity of symptoms. It's important to start with a low dose and slowly increase it until the desired results are achieved.

There are many potential benefits of CBD for animals, such as relieving anxiety, pain, inflammation, and skin issues. CBD can also help improve the overall health and well-being of pets. Some pet owners report that CBD has helped their pets sleep better and relax.

However, it's important to note that CBD may not be suitable for all pets and may have interactions with other medications the animal is taking. It's important to speak with a veterinarian before using CBD for your own pet.

Overall, CBD can be a promising option for improving the health and well-being of pets. If you're considering using CBD for your pet, it's important to educate yourself first and speak with a veterinarian to ensure it is safe and appropriate.

CBD and Pain in Animals

When it comes to pain in animals, it can be difficult to know how to help. Pain can be caused by various factors such as inflammation, injury, or disease. While there are veterinarians who prescribe pain medication, these drugs can have unwanted side effects. Fortunately, there is a natural alternative in the form of CBD.

CBD can alleviate pain in various ways. One of the main mechanisms is by reducing inflammation, which often causes pain. CBD can also help reduce pain perception by acting on the endocannabinoid system (ECS) in the animal's body. The ECS is a complex network of receptors and messengers that regulate various functions in the body, including pain perception and inflammatory responses.

CBD can be administered in various ways to alleviate pain in animals. One way is to use CBD oil, which can be given directly in the animal's mouth or added to their food. There are also topical CBD creams that can be applied to the affected area. Another advantage of CBD is that it has a high safety profile and is non-addictive, unlike many prescription pain medications.

It is important to note that the proper dosage of CBD is crucial to achieve maximum efficacy and minimal side effects. It is advisable to start with low doses and gradually increase the dosage until the optimal dose is found. It is recommended to consult with a veterinarian experienced with CBD to determine the right dosage for the specific animal and condition.

Overall, CBD is a promising option for alleviating pain in animals, particularly for those suffering from age, disease, or injury. With its anti-inflammatory and pain-relieving properties, CBD can be a safe and natural alternative to conventional pain medications.

CBD and Anxiety in Animals

CBD has also proven useful for pets suffering from anxiety. Anxiety in animals can have many causes, including bad experiences, separation anxiety, or even environmental changes like a move or a new pet in the house. When an animal suffers from anxiety, it can lead to unwanted behaviors such as aggression, inappropriate elimination, hyperactivity, and even self-injury. Fortunately, CBD can be a safe and natural way to treat anxiety in animals.

How does CBD work for anxiety in animals?

As with humans, CBD interacts with the endocannabinoid system of animals. This system helps maintain balance in the body and regulates important processes such as pain perception, appetite, and mood. By influencing the endocannabinoid system, CBD can help improve an animal's mood and behavior.

CBD can also help alleviate anxiety symptoms by reducing the level of the stress hormone cortisol. In chronic stress and anxiety disorders, cortisol is often present in excess, leading to overstimulation of the body. CBD can lower cortisol production, thereby reducing the body's stress response.

What do the studies say about the use of CBD in animals?

There are more and more scientific studies examining the use of CBD in animals. A study from 2019 examined the effects of CBD on dogs with anxiety related to noise. The results showed that CBD significantly improved the behavior of the dogs by reducing the number of barking dogs and lowering the heart rate of the animals.

Another study from 2018 examined the effects of CBD on cats with anxiety triggered by a change in their environment. The results showed that CBD improved the behavior of the cats by reducing the number of symptoms, including inappropriate elimination, inactivity, and aggression.

How can I use CBD on my pet?

It is important to always consult with a veterinarian before using CBD on a pet to ensure that there are no interactions with other medications and that the right dosage is chosen. There are different forms of CBD that can be used for animals, including oils, treats, and capsules. Oils can be given directly in the pet's food or applied to the fur, while treats and capsules can be used as snacks or mixed in with food.

CBD and sleep in pets

When it comes to our furry friends, we are always looking for ways to improve their health and well-being. And when it comes to sleep problems in animals, CBD can be a promising option.

CBD works on the endocannabinoid system, which is also present in animals and plays a role in regulating various bodily functions. In addition, CBD can also reduce inflammation and relieve pain, which can help animals feel more relaxed and sleep better.

Some pet owners have used CBD to treat sleep disorders in their pets and have seen positive results. For example, if an animal is anxious or in pain, which is affecting its sleep, CBD can help alleviate these symptoms and help it sleep more peacefully.

If you want to give your pet CBD, it's important to find an appropriate dosage. The dosage depends on various factors, such as the size of the animal, its weight, and the severity of its symptoms. It's also important to talk to a veterinarian before giving your pet CBD to ensure that it's safe and appropriate.

There are various ways to administer CBD to animals, such as oils, treats, and capsules. Some animals prefer one form over another, so it may require some trial and error to find out what works best for your pet.

While CBD is considered safe and effective for many animals, there are some factors to consider when using CBD in animals. For example, some animals may have an adverse reaction to CBD, especially if they take too much. It's important to increase the dosage slowly and carefully monitor the animal to ensure that there are no negative effects.

In summary, CBD can be a promising option for pet owners who want to help their pets sleep better. However, if you want to give CBD to your pet, it's important to talk to a veterinarian and find an appropriate dosage.

CBD and Other Health Conditions in Animals

CBD can not only help with pain and anxiety in animals, but there are also many other health problems where CBD may be a potential treatment option. In this chapter, I will explain some of these applications in more detail.

Some of the other health problems where CBD may be helpful include:

Inflammation: CBD has anti-inflammatory properties that can help treat inflammation in the bodies of animals. This can be especially beneficial in chronic inflammation, such as arthritis or inflammatory bowel disease.

Seizures: CBD has anticonvulsant properties and can therefore be helpful in treating seizures in animals, including epilepsy. There are some promising studies that suggest CBD may be an effective alternative to traditional medication.

Cancer: There are some promising research results that suggest CBD may help treat cancer in animals. One study showed that CBD inhibited the growth of breast cancer cells in mice. While further research is needed in this area, the results are promising.

Skin problems: CBD can also be helpful in treating skin problems in animals, such as allergic reactions, skin inflammation, or itching. CBD can be applied both orally and topically and has anti-inflammatory properties that can help with the treatment of skin problems.

Nausea and vomiting: CBD may be helpful in treating nausea and vomiting in animals, particularly when caused by chemotherapy or other medical treatments.

However, it is important to note that further research is needed in these areas to confirm the effectiveness of CBD in treating these health problems in animals. It is also important to always consult with a veterinarian before giving your pet CBD to ensure it is safe and appropriate.

Overall, there are many different applications of CBD in animals that go beyond pain and anxiety. While research in some of these areas is limited, the results are promising and it is possible that CBD may play an important role in veterinary medicine in the future.

Dosage and Safety in Use

When it comes to using CBD for animals, it is important to consider the proper dosage and safety. There are several important factors to consider before starting to use CBD for animals. In this chapter, I will tell you everything about the proper dosage and safety in using CBD for animals.

Firstly, it is important to note that animals may react differently to CBD than humans. Some animals may require higher or lower doses than others, depending on their size, weight, and individual response to CBD. It is also important to note that different animal species may require different dosages.

Before starting to use CBD for your pet, you should always speak with your veterinarian. Your veterinarian can help determine the right dosage for your animal and can also assist in monitoring for possible side effects.

There are various ways to administer CBD to animals, including CBD oils, capsules, treats, and topical creams. Each of these methods requires a different dosage, and it is important to follow the manufacturer's instructions carefully.

When using CBD oil, you should shake the bottle well before each use to ensure that the CBD is evenly distributed in the oil. You should also make sure that you are using the exact amount of oil recommended for the dosage.

With CBD treats, it is important to make sure that you are using the right amount recommended for the size of your pet. If using CBD capsules, you should make sure to open the capsule and mix the CBD powder with your pet's food.

It is also important to monitor for possible side effects when using CBD for your pet. Possible side effects of CBD for animals may include drowsiness, dry mouth, decreased blood pressure, and digestive issues.

It is important to be cautious when using CBD for your pet and to slowly increase the dosage to ensure that your pet does not experience any unwanted side effects.

If you notice any side effects, you should stop using CBD immediately and consult with your veterinarian.

In summary, dosage and safety in using CBD for animals are of great importance. It is important to follow the dosage carefully and monitor for possible side effects. Before starting to use CBD for your pet, you should always speak with your veterinarian and make sure to follow the manufacturer's instructions carefully.

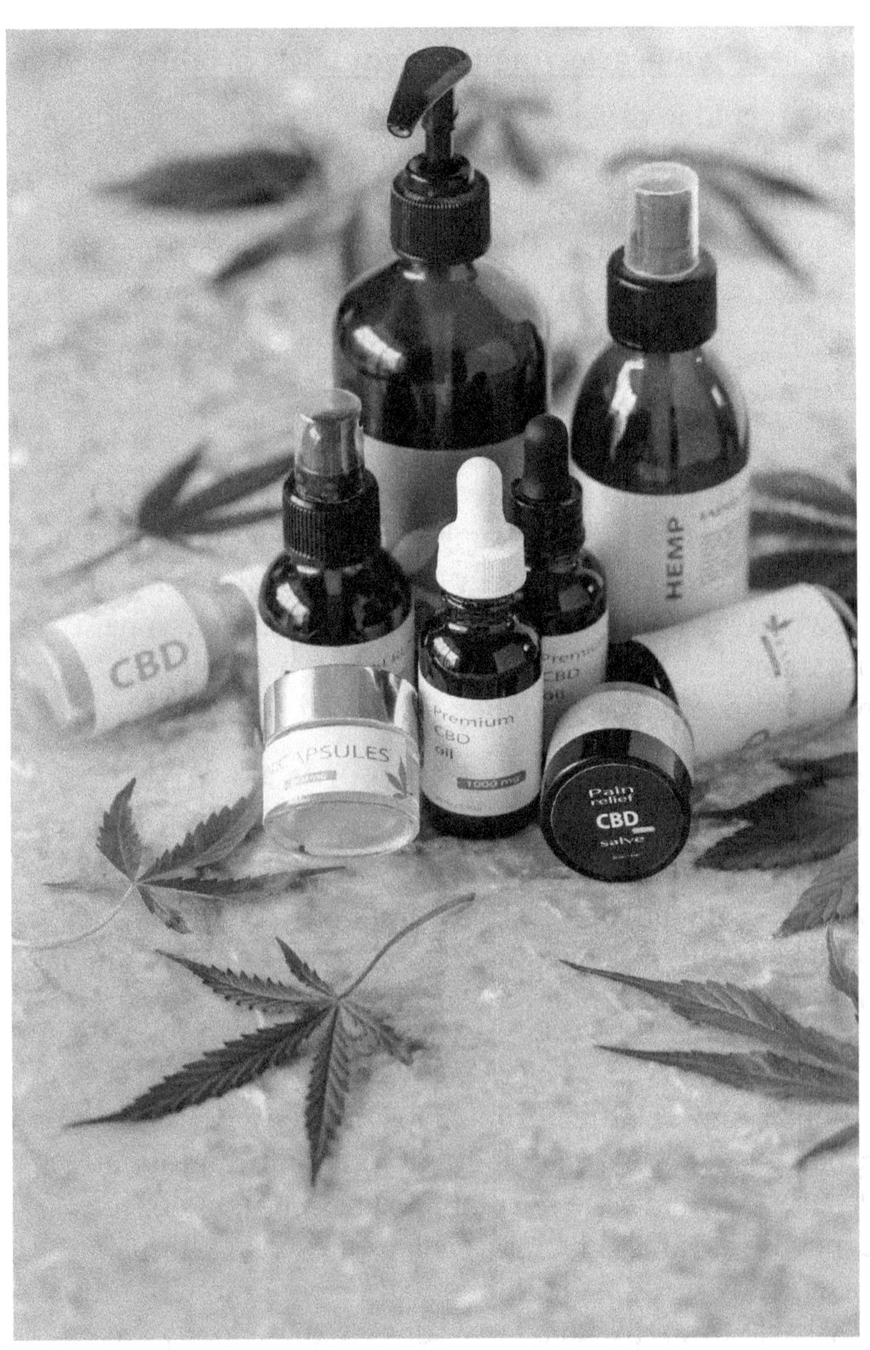
CBD
CAPSULES
Premium
CBD
oil
Premium
CBD
oil
1000 mg
HEMP
Pain
relief
CBD
salve

How to choose the right CBD product?

<u>Introduction to selecting the right CBD product.</u>

CBD is sold in different forms and concentrations, which can make it difficult to choose the right product. Choosing the right product depends on various factors, such as the reason for using CBD, the type of CBD product, and the dosage required. In this chapter, I will explain some important factors that you should consider when choosing the right CBD product.

Firstly, you should consider the reason for using CBD. If you want to take CBD to support your general health and well-being, you can consider using CBD oil or capsules. However, if you have specific complaints, such as pain, inflammation, or sleep problems, you may want to use a product specifically designed for these complaints.

It is also important to consider the type of CBD product. There are different types of CBD products, such as oils, capsules, tinctures, salves, and creams. Each type of product has its own advantages and disadvantages, and it may take a while to find the product that best suits you.

Another important factor in choosing the right CBD product is dosage. It is important to find an appropriate dosage to achieve the desired results. The right dosage depends on various factors, such as the reason for using CBD, body weight, and individual response to CBD. It is advisable to start with a lower dose and gradually increase it to determine how your body reacts to it.

Another important factor in choosing the right CBD product is the quality of the product. There are many low-quality CBD products on the market, so it is important to choose a high-quality product from a reputable manufacturer. Make sure that the product is made from hemp that has been grown according to organic standards and that it has been tested for quality and purity by an independent laboratory.

It is also important to consider the legislation in your country or region regarding CBD. CBD products are illegal in some countries or regions, while they are legal in others but may be subject to strict regulations. Make sure that the product you choose is legal and safe in your country or region.

CBD Isolate vs Full Spectrum CBD

CBD isolate and full spectrum CBD are two of the most commonly used types of CBD products on the market. Both have different pros and cons, and it is important to understand the differences between them in order to choose the right product for your specific needs.

CBD isolate is a concentrated form of pure CBD, where all other components of the hemp plant, including THC, have been removed. It is often sold as a white powder or crystals and is usually tasteless and odorless. CBD isolate is very versatile and can be used in different forms, such as tinctures, capsules, or in food and drinks.

Full spectrum CBD, on the other hand, contains a wider range of compounds from the hemp plant, including other cannabinoids like THC, terpenes, and flavonoids. These compounds work together to produce what's called the entourage effect, where they act synergistically and may be more effective than isolated CBD products. Full spectrum CBD is often available as oil and can also be used in tinctures, capsules, or topicals.

It is important to note that full spectrum CBD products may have psychoactive effects due to the presence of THC in small amounts. These effects are usually mild, but it is important to consider local laws, as the THC content may vary from product to product.

The choice between CBD isolate and full spectrum CBD depends on your specific needs and preferences. If you are sensitive to THC or need safe CBD products, CBD isolate may be the better choice. However, if you want to experience the potentially stronger effects of full spectrum CBD and THC use is legal in your country, this could be a good option.

CBD Oil vs. CBD Capsules vs. CBD Topicals

CBD oil, CBD capsules, and CBD topicals are three of the most popular CBD products on the market. Each has its own advantages and disadvantages, and the choice of the right product depends on your needs and preferences. In this chapter, I will help you understand the differences between CBD oil, CBD capsules, and CBD topicals so that you can make an informed decision.

CBD oil is the most well-known and popular CBD product. It is made by diluting CBD extract with a carrier oil such as hemp seed oil, olive oil, or coconut oil. CBD oil is usually dripped under the tongue and absorbed through the mucous membranes. It can also be mixed into food or beverages. CBD oil has the advantage of working quickly and being easy to dose. It can also be found in various concentrations and flavors to meet the needs and preferences of users.

CBD capsules are a convenient and discreet way to consume CBD. They contain a precisely dosed amount of CBD and are taken orally, similar to other dietary supplements or medications. CBD capsules are ideal for those who do not like the taste of CBD oil or who want to control the dosage more precisely. The disadvantage of CBD capsules is that they take longer to work as they have to go through the digestive tract before entering the bloodstream.

CBD topicals or topical products are another option for using CBD. These products are applied to the skin and can be used to relieve pain, inflammation, and skin problems such as eczema or acne. CBD topicals are also ideal for local application to joint or muscle pain. The advantage of topical products is that they can be applied specifically to certain areas of the body and do not have a systemic effect. The disadvantage is that they typically contain a lower concentration of CBD than oils or capsules, which makes them less effective for relieving stress and anxiety.

Ultimately, the choice between CBD oil, CBD capsules, and CBD topicals depends on your specific needs and preferences. If you want a quick effect, CBD oil may be the best option. If you need a precisely dosed amount of CBD, capsules are ideal. If you have pain or inflammation in a specific area, a topical application may be best. It is important to also pay attention to the concentration of the CBD product and ensure that it comes from a reputable manufacturer and has been tested for purity and quality by an independent entity.

Quality and Purity of CBD Products

When it comes to CBD products, the quality and purity of the product are crucial to ensuring that you are getting a safe and effective product. In this chapter, I will explain some important factors to consider when evaluating the quality and purity of CBD products.

Firstly, it is important to understand that the manufacturing of CBD products is crucial in ensuring a safe and high-quality product. There are various methods for extracting CBD from the hemp plant, and each method has its own advantages and disadvantages. One of the most effective and safest methods is CO2 extraction, which is a high-quality and pure method of CBD extraction.

Another factor that can influence the quality of CBD products is the type of hemp plant from which the CBD is extracted. It is important that the CBD is extracted from a hemp plant that has been sustainably grown and is free from pesticides and other harmful chemicals. There are many companies that specialize in growing high-quality hemp for CBD products, and it is important to purchase products from these trusted companies.

In addition to the type of hemp plant and extraction method, the purity of the CBD extract is also crucial. A high-quality CBD extract should be free from impurities such as heavy metals, pesticides, and other harmful chemicals. It is important that the company from which you are purchasing your CBD product provides independent lab results that confirm the purity and quality of the product.

Another factor to consider when evaluating the quality of CBD products is the type of carrier oils or ingredients used in the product. Some companies use low-quality carrier oils or ingredients that can compromise the quality of the product. It is important that the company from which you are purchasing your CBD product uses high-quality carrier oils and ingredients to ensure that the product is safe and effective.

In summary, when purchasing CBD products, it is important to pay attention to the quality and purity of the product. A high-quality CBD extraction method, sustainably grown hemp plant, independent lab results confirming the purity and quality of the product, as well as high-quality carrier oils and ingredients, are all important factors to consider in ensuring that you are getting a safe and effective CBD product.

Lab tests of CBD products

When it comes to buying CBD products, it is very important to ensure that the products are of the highest quality and purity. One way to ensure this is through lab testing.

In this chapter, I will explain to you what lab tests are, what types of tests are performed, and how you can ensure that the products you purchase have been tested.

Lab tests are an important method for verifying the quality and purity of CBD products. Through these tests, it can be determined whether the products are free from contaminants such as pesticides, heavy metals, and other impurities. They can also help determine the concentration of CBD and other cannabinoids in the product.

There are different types of lab tests that can be performed to determine the quality and purity of CBD products. Some of the most common tests are:

Potency tests: These tests determine the concentration of CBD and other cannabinoids in the product. They ensure that the product contains the concentration indicated on the packaging.

Pesticide tests: These tests ensure that the product is free from pesticides.

Heavy metal tests: These tests ensure that the product is free from heavy metals such as lead, mercury, and cadmium.

Solvent residue tests: These tests ensure that the product is free from solvent residues such as butane and ethanol, which can be used in the extraction of CBD.

It is important to ensure that the CBD products you buy have been tested through lab tests. This gives you the assurance that the product is of high quality and purity and does not contain harmful substances.

You should always look for CBD products that have been tested by independent labs. These labs should be accredited by an independent third party to ensure that the results are reliable.

If you want to see lab tests for a particular CBD product, you should contact the manufacturer and request a copy of the test results. Reputable manufacturers will be happy to share these results to validate their products.

Legality of CBD Products

In relation to CBD products, the question of legality is an important aspect. It is understandable that some people may have concerns when it comes to using CBD products. In this chapter, I will explain in detail what rules and regulations apply to CBD products and what this means for you and your furry friend.

Firstly, it should be clear that CBD products are legal in many countries. However, there are still restrictions or bans on CBD products in some countries. It is important to know the laws and regulations of your country or state before purchasing or using CBD products.

In most countries where CBD products are legal, there are restrictions regarding the THC content. THC is the psychoactive component of cannabis responsible for the "high" sensation. However, most CBD products contain only very low levels of THC that do not exceed the legal limit. In many countries, the legal limit for THC in CBD products is 0.3%. It is important to note that the legal regulations regarding THC limits can vary depending on the country or state.

In some countries, it is legal to buy and use CBD products, but not necessarily legal to sell them. In other countries, the sale of CBD products is legal as long as they comply with legal regulations. Therefore, it is important to know the laws of your country or state before purchasing or selling CBD products.

In some countries, CBD products are only available by prescription. This means that you must consult a veterinarian to obtain a prescription for CBD products. In other countries, you can buy CBD products without a prescription. However, it is important to note that the quality and purity of CBD products that are available without a prescription may not be as high as those of prescription products.

In some countries, there are also restrictions on the use of CBD products in animals. In these countries, it may be illegal to use CBD products in animals or there may be restrictions on the dosage or type of products that can be used. Therefore, it is important to know the laws of your country or state before applying CBD products to your pet.

It is also important to note that the legality of CBD products can change. Therefore, it is advisable to regularly inform yourself about the current laws and regulations regarding CBD products.

How to use CBD effectively?

Introduction to Using CBD

CBD is a versatile natural product with many potential health benefits and is becoming increasingly popular. In this chapter, I will give you an introduction to using CBD so that you can find the right dosage and the right products for your needs.

CBD is derived from the hemp plant and is a naturally occurring cannabinoid that acts on the body's endocannabinoid system. The endocannabinoid system is a complex network of receptors and neurotransmitters that plays an important role in regulating various physiological processes in the body, including pain perception, inflammation, mood, and sleep.

There are many different ways to consume CBD, including oils, capsules, gummies, topicals, and more. Each type of product has its own advantages and disadvantages, depending on why you want to take CBD and what kind of effect you want to achieve.

CBD oils are one of the most popular ways to consume CBD because they are a quick and effective method of getting CBD into the body. These oils are usually diluted in a carrier fluid like hemp seed oil or coconut oil and can be either placed directly in the mouth or mixed into food or drinks. CBD oils are also available in different concentrations so that you can precisely tailor the dosage to your needs.

CBD capsules are another popular option because they offer an easy way to consume CBD in a pre-defined dosage. Capsules are discreet and can be easily stored in a pill box, making them convenient to take on-the-go.

CBD gummies are a fun and delicious way to consume CBD and are often offered in various flavors and dosages. These gummies are well-suited for those who want to take CBD in a pleasant and easy-to-dose form.

CBD topicals like creams, lotions, and salves are ideal for local application on the skin or on affected areas to relieve pain or inflammation. Topicals can also help alleviate skin problems such as acne or eczema.

It is important to note that the effects of CBD can vary from person to person and that there is no "right" dosage. The optimal dosage depends on many factors, including your body weight, individual tolerance, and the type of CBD product you are using. It is recommended to start with a low dose and observe the effect before increasing the dose.

Overall, the use of CBD is an exciting and promising way to treat and alleviate various health problems.

The use of CBD flowers has several advantages over other CBD products. One of the main advantages is the quick effect. When smoking or vaporizing CBD flowers, the CBD is quickly absorbed into the lungs and quickly enters the bloodstream. This means that the effect can start within minutes and be quickly noticeable.

CBD flowers can be consumed in various ways. The most common method is smoking or vaporizing the flowers. However, if you do not want to smoke or vaporize, there are also other ways to consume CBD flowers. For example, you can add them to food or drinks to enjoy a CBD-rich meal.

Dosage of CBD

The dosage of CBD depends on many factors, such as individual body weight, the reason for taking CBD, the type of product, and the strength of the CBD extract. It is important to monitor the dosage carefully to achieve the best results.

As a general guideline, I recommend starting with a low dosage and gradually increasing it until the desired results are achieved. For adults, a typical starting dose of 10-20 mg of CBD per day is appropriate. This dose can be increased to up to 50-100 mg per day, depending on individual needs and tolerability.

When using CBD oil, it is important to consider the milligram strength of the product. A typical 30 ml bottle of 1000 mg CBD oil contains 33.3 mg of CBD per milliliter. For example, if you want to take 20 mg of CBD per day, you will need about 0.6 ml (approximately 12 drops) of the oil.

If you are new to using CBD, I recommend starting with lower strengths and gradually increasing the dosage until the desired results are achieved. It is also important to follow the manufacturer's instructions and not exceed the recommended dosage.

It is also worth noting that the type of CBD application can affect the dosage. When taking CBD oil sublingually (under the tongue), the CBD is absorbed more quickly into your body than when using CBD capsules or CBD foods. If you apply a product topically to your skin, a higher dosage may be necessary to achieve the same results as oral consumption.

Pregnancy and breastfeeding are times when it is best to avoid CBD as there is not enough research to ensure the safety of CBD during these times. Individuals who are taking blood-thinning medications should also be cautious and discuss the use of CBD with their doctor as CBD may interact with these medications.

Overall, it is important to start with a low dose and gradually increase the dosage to achieve the best results with CBD. It is also important to follow the manufacturer's instructions and not exceed the recommended dosage. If you have questions about the dosage of CBD, consult your doctor or a qualified CBD expert.

Using CBD Oil

CBD oil is one of the most popular forms of CBD products on the market, offering a variety of health and wellness benefits. In this chapter, I want to give you an introduction to using CBD oil and how it can help your body.

First of all, it's important to understand what CBD oil actually is. CBD oil is an extract made from the hemp plant. It contains cannabidiol (CBD) as well as other compounds that occur in the hemp plant, such as other cannabinoids, terpenes, and flavonoids.

CBD oil is often used as a dietary supplement to promote overall well-being. It can also be used to relieve pain, inflammation, anxiety, sleep disorders, and other health issues.

If you want to use CBD oil, there are some important factors to consider to ensure that you get the best results. Here are some steps to follow when using CBD oil:

Find the right dosage: The dosage of CBD oil depends on various factors, such as your body weight, body chemistry, and the severity of your symptoms. It's important to start with a low dosage and gradually increase until you find the optimal dosage for you.

Choose the right oil: There are different types of CBD oil that differ in their composition. There are full-spectrum CBD oils that contain other cannabinoids and terpenes in addition to CBD, as well as CBD isolates that only contain pure CBD. Depending on your individual needs and preferences, you should choose the right oil.

Check the purity and quality of the oil: It's important to use only high-quality CBD oils that have been tested for purity and quality. Look for brands that have their products tested by independent labs and whose results are publicly available.

Take the oil properly: CBD oil can be taken in various ways, such as directly under the tongue, in capsule or pill form, or by mixing it with food or drinks. You should choose the method that works best for you and make sure to dose the oil correctly.

Be patient and consistent: CBD oil may take some time to take effect. You should be patient and take the oil consistently to achieve the best results.

In summary, CBD oil is a useful and versatile product that can help improve your overall well-being. If you want to use CBD oil, you should make sure to follow these guidelines.

Using CBD Capsules

CBD capsules are a great alternative to CBD oil if you don't like the taste of hemp or prefer a discreet way to consume CBD. CBD capsules contain a precisely dosed amount of CBD in each capsule, making dosing and usage easier. In this chapter, I will explain everything you need to know about using CBD capsules.

Most CBD capsules are vegan and contain no artificial colors or flavors. They usually consist of CBD extract, carrier oil, and a capsule shell made of plant cellulose. The capsules are usually available in different dosages to meet individual needs.

Using CBD capsules is very simple. You simply take the desired number of capsules with water. The dosage varies depending on the person and symptoms. However, it is recommended to start with a low dosage and gradually increase it until you achieve the desired results. Note that it may take some time for the effects of CBD capsules to become noticeable, so give your body time to react to the CBD.

It is also important to note that CBD capsules should be taken on an empty stomach as this increases the absorption of CBD. If you take the capsules after a meal, the effect may be delayed or weakened.

CBD capsules are particularly suitable for people who need an accurate dosage or prefer a discreet way to consume CBD. They are also ideal for people who are on the go or don't have time to drop oil under their tongue.

As with all CBD products, you should ensure that you buy high-quality CBD capsules. Look for products that have been tested by third parties and have published results of those tests. Also, research the company that makes the capsules and choose a company that is transparent about its manufacturing processes and ingredients.

Overall, CBD capsules are a convenient, discreet, and accurate way to consume CBD. If you want to try CBD but don't like the taste of hemp oil or prefer an easy way to dose CBD, CBD capsules are a great option.

Use of CBD flowers

CBD flowers have gained popularity in recent years and are now used by many people as an alternative to CBD oil or capsules. However, unlike other CBD products, CBD flowers are not legal in all countries and it is important to comply with local laws and regulations.

CBD flowers are derived from hemp plants that have been specifically bred for their high CBD content. They also contain other cannabinoids, terpenes, and flavonoids that can together create the so-called entourage effect. The entourage effect describes the synergistic effect of the different ingredients that can contribute to a stronger and more effective effect.

CBD flowers can be consumed in various ways, including smoking, vaporizing, and preparing as a tea. Smoking CBD flowers is the most common method and can be done quickly and easily. However, smoking flowers can also have some disadvantages, especially for people with respiratory diseases. An alternative is vaporizing, in which the flowers are heated in a vaporizer and the vapor is inhaled. Vaporizing is usually gentler on the lungs and can also allow for more effective absorption of CBD.

CBD flowers can also be prepared as tea by soaking them in hot water. This method can have a gentler effect, as CBD is released more slowly and the body has more time to absorb it. In addition, drinking CBD tea can have a calming and relaxing effect, which is particularly popular among people with stress or anxiety.

When using CBD flowers, it is important to pay attention to quality and purity. It is advisable to only buy products from reputable manufacturers who test their products in independent laboratories to ensure they are free of pollutants and contaminants. It is also important to pay attention to the dosage and start with a small amount to test the body's reaction.

Overall, the use of CBD flowers can be an effective and natural way to benefit from the potential health benefits of CBD. However, if you decide to use CBD flowers, it is important to find the right method and dosage to achieve the best possible results.

Combination of CBD

CBD can be taken in various ways, and it is also possible to combine it with other substances. Such a combination can enhance or complement the effects of CBD, and potentially even reduce the dosage required. In this chapter, I will give you an overview of some common combinations of CBD with other substances.

CBD and Hemp:

One of the most obvious combinations of CBD is with

hemp. Hemp not only contains CBD but also many other cannabinoids, terpenes, and flavonoids that can achieve a synergistic effect when combined. This is known as the "entourage effect," meaning that the effects of CBD are amplified or improved when combined with other hemp components.

It is important to note that hemp products may contain a low amount of THC, which has psychoactive effects and is illegal in some countries. If you want to use hemp products, you should ensure they meet the legal requirements in your country and consider the risk of THC consumption.

CBD and Caffeine:

Many people combine CBD and caffeine as they believe that CBD can help reduce the excitement and nervousness caused by caffeine. However, there is no sufficient scientific evidence to prove that this combination produces a better effect than caffeine or CBD alone. Some studies have shown that CBD can modulate the effects of caffeine on the central nervous system.

CBD and Alcohol:

CBD is often considered a way to mitigate the effects of alcohol. Combining CBD and alcohol can lead to an enhanced effect of CBD and a reduced alcohol high. However, it is important to note that both alcohol and CBD have sedative effects, and combining these two substances can lead to increased sedation.

CBD and Nicotine:

CBD and nicotine can be combined to mitigate the effects of nicotine. CBD can also help reduce withdrawal symptoms during smoking cessation. However, it is important to note that smoking is harmful to health, and the combination of CBD and nicotine does not fully eliminate the harmful effects of smoking.

CBD and Other Medications:

If you are already taking medication, you should consult your doctor before taking CBD, as CBD can influence the effects of other medications. For example, CBD can inhibit the breakdown of drugs in the liver, which can enhance the effects of these medications. This can lead to unwanted side effects.

CBD in sports

How CBD can improve your athletic performance

Sport is a great way to improve your health, but it can also be demanding and take a toll on your body. It is important to take care of your body and support it in order to increase your athletic performance and avoid injuries. One way to do this is by using CBD.

CBD has many potential benefits for athletes and fitness enthusiasts. A 2018 study published in the Journal of Sports Medicine and Physical Fitness found that CBD can accelerate recovery after exercise and reduce inflammation. There is also evidence that CBD can alleviate pain and improve sleep quality, which is crucial for post-workout recovery.

Another way in which CBD can improve your athletic performance is its ability to enhance focus. CBD can reduce stress and anxiety, which can help you concentrate on your training and better focus on your goals.

Another benefit of CBD is its ability to lower blood pressure. A 2017 study published in the Journal of Clinical Investigation found that CBD can lower blood pressure, which can be particularly beneficial for athletes. High blood pressure can cause the heart to work harder to pump enough oxygen to the muscles. By lowering your blood pressure, CBD can help your

heart work more efficiently and transport more oxygen to the muscles.

CBD can also help improve muscle recovery. A 2015 study published in the Free Radical Biology and Medicine Journal found that CBD has an antioxidant effect and can therefore help reduce the damage caused by free radicals during exercise. This can help the muscles recover more quickly and prepare more quickly for the next workout.

There is also evidence that CBD can help improve lung function. A 2015 study published in the Frontiers in Pharmacology Journal found that CBD can help improve bronchodilation, which can be beneficial for athletes who suffer from asthma or have difficulty breathing.

If you want to use CBD to improve your athletic performance, there are various ways to take it. CBD oil, capsules, and flowers can all be helpful, depending on your preferences and which method is best suited for your needs. However, it is important to follow dosage recommendations and ensure that you use high-quality, safe products.

Overall, there are many good reasons why you should incorporate CBD into your fitness routine.

CBD and Pain Relief in Sports

I would be happy to give you an overview of how CBD can help with pain relief in sports. CBD can help to reduce pain and inflammation, making it a promising dietary supplement for athletes.

CBD works on the endocannabinoid system (ECS) in the body, which is responsible for regulating pain, inflammation, and various other functions. It can help the pain receptors of the ECS to reduce pain signals in the body.

Pain is often an indicator of inflammation in the body. If you experience pain and swelling after a strenuous workout or sporting event, CBD can help by reducing inflammation. CBD can also help improve muscle recovery and shorten the time it takes to recover from an injury.

Another advantage of CBD is that it is a natural remedy that has no unwanted side effects. Unlike prescription painkillers or anti-inflammatory drugs, which can often have serious side effects, CBD is a natural, safe, and effective alternative.

If you decide to use CBD for pain relief, it is important to find the right dosage. The optimal dosage depends on various factors such as body weight, metabolism, and the severity of the pain. It is best to start with a lower dosage and gradually increase it until you find the optimal dosage.

CBD can be taken in various forms, such as oil, capsules, or topicals. Some athletes prefer topical application as it can be applied directly to the affected area. Others prefer oral ingestion of CBD as it is quickly absorbed by the body.

Overall, CBD can be a valuable addition for any athlete looking for a safe and effective method of pain relief and inflammation reduction. However, it is always important to speak with a doctor before taking CBD to ensure that there are no interactions with other medications and that it is safe for you.

CBD and Recovery After Exercise

After an intense workout, it's important to give your body the necessary time to recover in order to avoid injuries and pain, and improve your athletic performance. CBD can play a supportive role in this process.

One way to use CBD for recovery is through topical application. CBD creams and salves can be applied directly to affected areas to relieve pain and inflammation. CBD can also help promote the recovery of muscles and tissues by increasing blood flow and oxygen to affected areas.

Another approach is to use CBD oil, which can be taken orally or sublingually, under the tongue. This allows the CBD to be quickly absorbed into the bloodstream and target affected areas. CBD can help relieve pain and reduce inflammation, which can help the body recover and regenerate more quickly.

It's important to note that CBD alone is not enough to guarantee fast recovery. A healthy diet, adequate sleep, and rest are also crucial. Additionally, athletes should pay attention to appropriate training intensity and give themselves enough time to recover.

While there are many positive reports on the use of CBD for recovery, there are currently no comprehensive clinical studies confirming the effectiveness and safety of CBD for post-workout recovery. Therefore, it's important to consult with a qualified physician or other medical professional before using CBD.

In summary, CBD presents a promising option for supporting recovery after exercise. It can help relieve pain and inflammation, and increase blood flow and oxygen, which can contribute to faster recovery. However, it's important to consider CBD as part of a holistic approach to recovery and to consult with a qualified physician or other medical professional before use.

CBD and stress reduction in sports

Sports can be a great way to reduce stress. However, there may be times when your stress levels are high, such as in competitive situations or when you are focused on a goal. In such cases, CBD can be a useful supplement.

Stress can be both physical and mental and can lead to a variety of symptoms that can affect your athletic performance. These include muscle tension, sleep disorders, anxiety, nervousness, and exhaustion. CBD can help alleviate these symptoms and thus reduce your stress.

CBD can also help reduce muscle tension, which is often caused by stress. By increasing blood flow and oxygen to the muscles, it can help the muscles relax and recover.

In addition, CBD can help treat sleep disorders, which are often caused by stress. When you're stressed, it can be difficult to fall asleep or stay asleep at night. CBD can help regulate your sleep cycle and improve your sleep quality.

Finally, CBD can also help alleviate anxiety and nervousness, which are often associated with stressful situations. It can help you stay calm and focused, even when you're under pressure.

How to use CBD for sports - Dosage, administration, and recommendations

CBD has the potential to improve your athletic performance, alleviate pain, promote recovery, and reduce stress. But how do you use CBD for sports?

In this chapter, I'll show you how to best use CBD for your athletic activities.

First of all, you should know that the dosage and administration of CBD are very individual. There is no general recommendation that applies to everyone. The right dosage depends on various factors, such as your body weight, your tolerance to CBD, the intensity of your athletic activities, and the desired effect.

If you're new to the world of CBD, you should start with a low dose and gradually increase it until you achieve the desired results. A typical dose for beginners is about 5-10 mg per day. If you already have experience with CBD, you can increase your dose to up to 50 mg per day. However, it's important not to take too much, as an overdose can have undesirable side effects.

CBD can be administered in various ways, including CBD oil, CBD capsules, CBD creams and ointments, and CBD flowers. The choice of the right administration form depends on your personal preferences and needs.

For example, if you need fast-acting results, CBD oils and capsules are a good choice as they are quickly absorbed by the body. CBD creams and ointments are a good choice if you have local pain or inflammation as they can be applied directly to the affected area. CBD flowers can be smoked or vaporized and are a good choice for people who don't like the taste of CBD oil.

There are also various CBD products specifically designed for athletes. These products may contain additional ingredients such as caffeine, B vitamins, and electrolytes that can help improve your athletic performance.

CBD and doping control in sports - Is CBD safe for athletes?

As an athlete, you want to ensure that you can take advantage of all the benefits that CBD can bring to your body and performance. But it's also important to know if CBD is safe for athletes and if it's allowed in doping controls. In this chapter, I want to give you all the important information about this.

First of all, it's important to understand that CBD is not the same as THC, which contains psychoactive compounds in marijuana. CBD is not psychoactive and does not have a intoxicating effect. That means you don't have to worry about any unwanted psychological effects when using CBD.

However, it's also important to know that CBD products are generally not tested in laboratories approved by the World Anti-Doping Agency (WADA). Although CBD itself is not a prohibited substance on the WADA list, there is always a risk that other substances in a CBD product may result in a positive doping test.

It's also possible that some CBD products may contain traces of THC that can be detected in doping tests. Although these traces are usually very low, depending on the amount of CBD you take, a positive doping test can occur.

This is an important point to consider when using CBD products in sports.

Why CBD can be a valuable supplement for athletes

First of all, it's important to understand that athletes are often subjected to significant physical stress that can lead to imbalances in their bodies. This is where CBD can come into play, as it can help restore the body's balance and support the body in coping with stress.

CBD can help improve physical performance by supporting the body's recovery, reducing pain, and decreasing inflammation in the body. Additionally, CBD can also help reduce stress and anxiety, which can be especially important for competitive athletes.

Another advantage of CBD as a supplement for athletes is that it provides a natural and gentle alternative to prescription drugs. While many athletes rely on medication to relieve pain or reduce inflammation, which is often associated with side effects, CBD offers a natural alternative without the risks and side effects that may accompany prescription drugs.

However, it's important to note that CBD is not a cure-all and cannot be solely responsible for an athlete's success. Instead, it should be viewed as part of a holistic approach to improving physical performance, which also includes aspects such as training, nutrition, and rest periods.

Conclusion

Summary of Key Findings

Congratulations, you made it to the end of my book! Before you return to your daily routine, I'd like to summarize the key findings of this book.

CBD is a natural compound derived from the hemp plant with diverse health-promoting properties. It can help alleviate pain, anxiety, sleep problems, and other health issues.

The use of CBD in sports is an emerging research area, and there is ample evidence that it can aid athletes in performance enhancement, recovery, and stress reduction.

CBD can be consumed in various forms, such as oils, capsules, creams, and flowers, and through different dosages and administration methods. It's important to find the right dosage and administration method for your individual needs and goals.

If you're an athlete and want to use CBD, make sure the product you're using is of high quality and free of THC. Additionally, you should educate yourself on the guidelines and regulations regarding the use of CBD in sports.

Overall, CBD is a promising supplement for athletes that can serve as a natural alternative to prescription medications. It can contribute to improving athletic performance, recovery, and stress reduction, and its health-promoting properties make it a valuable addition to a healthy lifestyle.

Outlook: What the Future Holds for CBD

Science is delving more and more into CBD and its potential benefits. In the future, we will likely learn much more about CBD and its effects on the human body.

A promising direction in CBD research is the investigation of its effects on specific sports activities. For example, CBD could be studied to see how it affects swim training or how it speeds up the recovery of runners. There are countless ways CBD could help athletes enhance their performance.

Another exciting area of CBD research is the examination of the role of CBD in relation to other cannabinoids and plant compounds, such as the well-known THC. In the past, CBD has often been associated with THC, but we now know that CBD offers a range of benefits independent of THC. But what happens when CBD is taken in combination with other compounds? What effects does that have on the body and athletic performance? These are questions we will hopefully find answers to in the future.

Another area in which CBD research is likely to advance is the investigation of the effects of CBD on various health conditions and diseases, such as depression, anxiety, and inflammation. Since these conditions are often associated with sports activities and performance, CBD could be a promising addition to traditional treatment methods.

Ultimately, there is still so much to discover and explore

when it comes to CBD and its effects on the body. One thing is certain, however: CBD has the potential to change the way we improve our athletic performance and optimize our health.

So, stay tuned and keep an eye out for further developments in the world of CBD. Who knows what surprises the future holds!

Thank you to the readers

Dear readers,

I want to express my heartfelt gratitude to you for taking the time to read my book on CBD and its potential. I hope that I was able to provide you with valuable insights and knowledge that will help you improve your performance and optimize your recovery.

It brings me great joy to share my knowledge and experience with you, and I hope that you have benefited from it. I am confident that CBD can be a valuable supplement for athletes, and that there will be many more insights and applications in the future.

I would love to hear from you and learn how you are using CBD in sports and what experiences you have had with it. Please feel free to send me an email or follow me on social media so that we can stay in touch.

Once again, thank you for reading my book, and I wish you all the best in your athletic activities and your health.

Best regards,

Rapha

Further Reading and Sources

In this chapter, I would like to recommend some additional sources and resources to deepen your knowledge about CBD in sports. There is a lot of information out there, and it can be difficult to figure out which sources are trustworthy and well-founded. That's why I have compiled some resources that I have used myself and found valuable.

Books:

"CBD: A Patient's Guide to Medicinal Cannabis" by Leonard Leinow and Juliana Birnbaum

"The Athlete's Guide to CBD: Treat Pain and Inflammation, Maximize Recovery, and Sleep Better Naturally" by Scott Douglas and Sarah Talansky

"The CBD Oil Miracle: Manage Pain, Improve Your Mood, Boost Your Brain, Fight Inflammation, Clear Your Skin, Strengthen Your Heart, and Sleep Better with the Healing Power of CBD Oil" by Laura Lagano

Scientific Articles:

"Cannabidiol and Sports Performance: a Narrative Review of Relevant Evidence and Recommendations for Future Research" by Matthew B. Jones and Zeke J. Walton

"Cannabidiol as a Potential Treatment for Anxiety Disorders" by Esther M. Blessing, Maria M. Steenkamp, Jorge Manzanares, and Charles R. Marmar

"Pharmacology of Cannabinoids in the Treatment of Epilepsy" by Orrin Devinsky, Maria Roberta Cilio, and Helen Cross

Websites:

Project CBD (https://www.projectcbd.org/)

Leafly (https://www.leafly.com/)

National Center for Complementary and Integrative Health (https://www.nccih.nih.gov/health/cannabis-marijuana-and-cannabinoids-what-you-need-to-know)

Please note that this is only a small selection of the available sources and that it is important to always remain critical and to verify the sources. It is also important to mention that research on CBD and its effects is still relatively young and that further studies are needed to fully understand its effectiveness and safety.

I hope this book has given you a good insight into the topic of CBD in sports and that you are now better informed when it comes to whether or not to use CBD as a dietary supplement. If you have any further questions or need more information, please do not hesitate to research additional sources or to consult an expert in this field.

Imprint

Pics by:

Nataliya Vaitkevich

AlesiaKozik

www.ingramcontent.com/pod-product-compliance
Lightning Source LLC
Chambersburg PA
CBHW061615250726
48653CB00018B/582